HOW TO DO THE KETOGENIC DIET WITHOUT STOPPING EATING

BURN YOUR BODY FAT IN THREE WEEKS IN A HEALTHY WAY, THE MOST EFFECTIVE DIET TO LOSE WEIGHT

Jessy M. Brown

Table of Contents

Introduction: Low-Carbohydrate Diet

To help with weight problems and to improve overall health, many people turn to dieting. In fact, government statistics show that while about 65 percent of Americans are overweight, 38 percent are doing something about it.

And according to a recent survey by the National Institutes of Health, about one-third of overweight Americans who are trying to lose weight are doing so by eating fewer carbohydrates largely because of the increased popularity of fad diets such as the Atkins diet and the South Beach diet.

Although there certainly have been

other low-carbohydrate or low-sugar diet plans before, and more likely to come out in the coming years, let's take a look at the fundamentals behind many of the major plans. And let's take a look at how they fit into today's real world. Because while it might be great to reduce your body's sugar content and be healthier, wouldn't it be great to learn how to do it while being part of this fast-paced world?

In the world of instant messaging, rapid interaction on the Internet and the already multifaceted and hectic daily schedules, dietary food budgeting, planning, preparation and shopping are topics that can become major sources of stress and reasons for diet failure. Moving double-income families and other super-employed wage earners and dieters often already suffer more from their share of everyday stressors such as fear of being fired, their jobs being relocated or terminated, juggling more than one job, dependents (both elderly and underage) and trying to finance and juggle with continuing education in their lives, budgets and daily routines.

People want and need simpler solutions. And they need simpler diet plans. Forget about spending large sums of money on hard-to-find gourmet items. Forget about spending hours just to prepare meals. And forget about counting, measuring and weighing the ingredients.

Either a low-carb plan fits into real life or it doesn't. We'll first take a look at some basic terms and definitions to help understand the science behind low-carbohydrate plans. Let's see how many of the players' main plans are up to the task.

Please note that the content here is not

presented by a physician, and that all dietary planning should be done under the guidance of your own physicians. This content only presents an overview of low-carbohydrate research for educational purposes and does not replace the medical advice of a professional physician.

Types of carbohydrates

Simply put, there are two types of carbohydrates, simple and complex. Some refer to them as bad and good carbohydrates, fast and slow digesting carbohydrates, and others as possibly confusing. Here's the scoop.

➤ Simple carbohydrates

-

Foods with simple or refined carbohydrates often have low nutrient content and a high glycaemic index. They are rapidly digested and can cause blood sugar to skyrocket and then fall dramatically in a short period of time. In order to keep the body functioning healthier and more stable, health advisors recommend that these types of foods be limited.

Examples of these simple carbohydrates are white bread, potatoes, bananas, and sugary treats such as cookies, candy, muffins, and cakes, and carbonated beverages such as popular cola products.

> ### ➢ *Complex carbohydrates*
-

Foods with complex carbohydrates contain many nutrients and have a low to moderate glycemic index. A higher fiber content in these foods means slower digestion, which is healthier for the body. And these foods are considered good choices by health advisors.

Examples of these complex carbohydrates are whole grains, most fruits and vegetables. Legumes, plants of the pea or bean family, are also in this category.

> ### ➢ *Which one's the best?*

While studies such as that of the University of Arkansas for Medical Sciences in January 2004 show that low-carbohydrate diets can help with weight loss; carbohydrates should be of the complex, low-glycemic index type. Remarkable is that a total avoidance of simple carbohydrates is not necessary, either. In other words, occasional treatment, in moderation (and approved by your dietary advisor or in agreement with your doctor), should be fine.

As a side note, your teeth will also be healthier without the build-up of sugar decay from simple carbohydrate foods. So that the healthiest smiles shine with healthier bodies.

Other concepts you should know

Here are some other terms that help explain the scientific and health problems behind low-carbohydrate dietary planning solutions. Please note that these are only basic definitions and can be explored in your spare time through other resources to better define your functions in the body's health system.

CALORIES

A calorie is a measure of heat. Calories also refer to a measure of the amount of energy a body gets from food. Simply put, the more calories in food, the more energy it takes for the body to use the nutrients.

CARBOHYDRATE

A carbohydrate is one of the three main nutrients that provide energy to the body. Carbohydrates are composed of simple sugars or linked sugar chains.

Examples of simple sugars (simple carbohydrates) are sucrose or table sugar, fructose or fruit sugar, and lactose or milk sugar. Tied chains of sugar or complex carbohydrates found in plants are often called starches.

Examples of digestible complex carbohydrate types are wheat flour or potato starch. An undigestible example is celery cellulose. Carbohydrates are converted by the body into sugar and used as energy. Unused carbohydrates are stored in the body as fat.

GREASE

Fat is one of the three main groups of nutrients that provide energy to the body. Fat is obtained from animal or vegetable oil sources. The body breaks it down into simpler fats and burns them or stores them in the body.

FRUCTOSE

Fructose is a plant-derived sugar, especially corn, which is used to sweeten commercial food products such as soft drinks and other prepared foods. Its popularity first spread in the 1970s and it is often listed as "high fructose corn syrup.

GLUCOSA

Glucose is known as blood sugar. All carbohydrates, whether simple or complex, are converted by the body into sugar and the sugar within the body's bloodstream is this way. The level of glucose in the blood is the main stimulus for insulin secretion.

GLUCAGON

Glucagon is a hormone produced by the pancreas that stimulates fat cells to convert their stores into glucose and release them for energy use. Glucagon must be released for the body to release and break down body fat. The pancreas cannot efficiently release both glucagon and insulin and will not release glucagon if blood sugar and insulin levels are high.

GLYCOGEN

Glycogen is the main form of carbohydrate storage in animals and is found mainly in the liver and muscle tissue. It is easily converted to glucose as needed by the body to meet its energy needs. Also called animal starch.

GLYCEMIC INDEX

The glycemic index is a measure of how quickly individual foods will raise your body's blood sugar level.

INSULIN

Insulin is one of the two main hormones produced by the pancreas and the body's main metabolic hormone. When blood glucose increases, the pancreas releases insulin to help transfer glucose to cells for energy.

Insulin also helps convert extra glucose into fatty tissue and helps promote amino acids that are converted into proteins and stored in muscle. In the liver, it helps the extra glucose to be stored as glycogen. Insulin can raise cholesterol levels and cause fluid and salt retention, and stands

in the way of breaking down stored fat.
Lack of adequate insulin or lack of
sufficient insulin

sensitivity to the effects of insulin on the
body can lead to diabetes.

INSULIN RESISTANCE

Insulin resistance is a condition that is
reached when the body does not respond
and properly processes the insulin it
releases. Insulin resistance causes the
pancreas to overproduce insulin.
According to Dr. Michael and Dr. Mary
Eades of Protein Power, insulin resistance
causes high blood pressure, elevated
cholesterol levels, coronary artery disease
(heart disease), obesity, type II diabetes,
and a host of other diseases and
disorders.

KETONES

When the body breaks down fat for energy due to a lack of enough glucose to meet energy needs, combined with the depletion of glycogen in the liver, ketones are a type of chemical result. Excess ketones cause bad breath and appear in the urine during the strip test.

CETOSIS

Ketosis is the body's process of burning stored fat for energy when glucose is not readily available. A survival mechanism used in times of famine.

It is generally thought that it is not a good long-term state for the body to operate on it. When ketosis occurs in someone who is a victim of famine, or who is not eating food for any reason, it can cause serious illness and eventually death.

PROTEIN

Protein is one of the three main groups of nutrients that provide energy to the body. Protein is made from animal and soy products and some vegetable products such as legumes (beans, peanuts and peas). Converted into amino acids by the body during digestion and stored in muscle cells as protein.

SUCROSE

Another name for sucrose is table sugar; it is derived from sugar cane plants.

STAR

Starch is a type of sugar found in potatoes, white rice, breads, bagels, and other foods.

TRANS GREASE

Trans fat is a type of processed fat that is not found in nature (also called hydrogenated or partially hydrogenated fat/oil). It is used in baked goods such as doughnuts, breads, crackers, chips, cookies and many other processed food products such as margarine and salad dressings.

A little bit of history: The start of the "low-carbohydrate" diet.

Low-carbohydrate" terminology was not really coined until around 1992 when the USDA announced that the U.S. model food pyramid included six to eleven daily servings of grains and starches. However, low-carbohydrate diets date back more than 100 years before Atkins' fad diet, to 1864, with a booklet titled Letter on Corpulence written by William Banting, as close as possible to the first commercial low-carbohydrate diet available.

Banting had suffered a series of debilitating health problems mainly due to his overweight or "corpulence". He searched in vain for cures for his weight problem, which many doctors at the time believed was a necessary side effect of old age. He also tried to eat less, but continued to gain weight and have several health problems. He couldn't understand how the small amounts of food he was eating led to his weight problem:

"Few men have led a more active life - bodily or mentally - of a constitutional anxiety for regularity, precision and order, for fifty years of my entrepreneurial career, from which I had retired, so that my corpulence and subsequent obesity were not due to carelessness of necessary bodily activity, nor by eating, drinking or excessive complacency of any kind, except that I took the simple foods of bread, milk, butter, beer, sugar and potatoes with more freedom than my age required.... of me.

Many contemporary Americans on the move may recognize Banting's unhealthy daily diet:

"My old diet table was bread and milk

for breakfast, or a pint of tea with lots of milk, sugar and toast with butter; meat, beer, lots of bread (which I was always very fond of) and pastries for dinner, tea lunch similar to breakfast, and usually a fruit cake or bread and milk for dinner. I had little comfort and much less deep sleep."

Just replace a cake, donut or muffin with coffee and lots of cream and sugar for breakfast, a fast-food burger and fries with a large soda for lunch and a frozen cake or pizza for dinner followed by dessert and you'll see how Banting's diet was so similar to that of today's fast-paced Americans.

When her doctor placed these items on a "Prohibited Food List," Banting lost 50 pounds and 13 inches in one year. He stayed away, living a long and much healthier life.

His new diet plan consisted of a series of

meat dishes and listed it as follows:

"For breakfast, at 9:00 a.m., I take five to six ounces of lamb, kidneys, roast fish, bacon, or cold meat of any kind, except pork or beef; a large cup of tea or coffee (without milk or sugar), a small cookie, or an ounce of dry toasted bread; making together six ounces of solid, nine ounces of liquid.

For dinner, at 14:00 hours, five or six ounces of any fish except salmon, herring,

or eels, any meat except pork or veal, any vegetable except potato, parsnip, beet, turnip or carrot, one ounce of dry toasted bread, fruit of a pudding that does not sweeten any type of poultry or game, and two or three glasses of good claret, sherry or Madeira, or champagne, port and beer prohibited; making together ten to twelve solid and ten fluid ounces.

For tea, at 6:00 p.m., two or three ounces of cooked fruit, one or two cookies, and a cup of tea without milk or sugar; making two to four solid ounces, nine fluid.

For dinner, 9:00 P.M. Three or four ounces of meat or fish, similar to dinner, with a glass or two of claret or sherry and water; making four solid ounces and seven liquid.

For the glass, if necessary, a glass of grog (gin, whisky or brandy, without sugar), or one or two glasses of claret or sherry".

So great were the changes in his appearance and health that his friends and acquaintances began to notice and just like today they wanted to know what diet he was following. The most important thing of all is that Banting could feel and see the difference for himself.

"Everyone who knows me tells me that my personal appearance has improved a lot and that I seem to bear the seal of good health; this may be a matter of opinion or a friendly comment, but I can honestly say that I feel restored to health, "bodily and mentally," that I seem to have more muscle strength and vigor, that I eat and drink with a good appetite, and that I sleep well. All symptoms of heartburn, indigestion, and heartburn (with which I was often tormented) have disappeared. I have stopped using starting hooks, and other aids such as these, which were indispensable but are now able to bend down easily and freely, are unnecessary. I have lost the feeling of occasional fainting, and what I think is a blessing and a remarkable consolation, is that I have been able to leave the knee pads, which I had necessarily used for many years, and that I have abandoned the umbilical bandage.

His book on dieting became very popular and was translated into several languages. However, it was eventually abandoned.

Banting pointed out in the Charter on Corpulence that a common health paradox of our time did not exist in his. This was the paradox of obesity, widely regarded as a problem of excess, among the poor. The poor of the 19th century could not afford the refined sugary foods that cause weight gain. But the poor of the 21st century can do it today.

In a recent Associated Press article titled "Health Paradox: Obesity Attacks the Poor," the reporter noted that many poor families are increasing their food budgets by buying unhealthy processed and refined foods. From a family that Barbassa wrote,

"During the winter, jobs are scarce, so Caballero feeds her husband and three children with the cheapest food she can get: potatoes, bread, tortillas.... Como is processed.

foods rich in sugar and fat have become cheaper than fruits and vegetables, the poor in particular are paying a high price with rates of obesity rising, followed by diabetes.

Unfortunately for the Caballero family, these cheap staples are bad for their health. Fresh meat, low starch fruits and vegetables may be more expensive and have a shorter shelf life, but they are definitely worth the price in saved medical expenses and better health.

Over the years, as "calories" became known, variations in calorie counts were included in dietary solutions. And a variety of other topics were explored such as how many of the foods should be consumed and how often.

As the Banting diet finally fell into disuse, low-carbohydrate diets began to reappear in the 20th century. The most famous are the Atkins and Scarsdale diets that became popular in the 1970s. While Scarsdale has a 14-day meal plan that must be followed and severely restricts calories, the Atkins diet allowed unlimited calorie intake as long as those calories come from protein, fat and vegetables and carbohydrate intake was kept low.

Atkins and Scarsdale fell out of favor in the 1980s when the U.S. Department of Agriculture encouraged the consumption of grains and grain products with the USDA food pyramid.

It was only in the 1990s that we began to see a return to low-carbohydrate diets that seem to be more than just a fad. It's a lifestyle! As more and more people realize the weight loss and other health benefits that are available to people who eat low-carbohydrates, the number of diets and stores that sell special low-carbohydrate products continues to increase.

In short, most low-carbohydrate diets have the same basic premise: that excess of simple, refined carbohydrates leads to overproduction of insulin, leading to the storage of too much fat in the body. This fat storage is especially prominent around the middle.

Although there are degrees of difference between the many diets, they all agree on the negative effects that excess insulin production has on our systems.

Insulin, what is its function?

There are three basic units that the body uses for energy:

> Fat
> Protein
> Carbohydrates

All three can be converted to blood glucose. However, while fats and proteins are converted slowly, carbohydrates are converted quickly causing rapid spikes in blood sugar levels in the body. These spikes in blood sugar levels cause the pancreas to create and release insulin until the blood sugar level returns to normal.

Meanwhile, insulin, a hormone produced in the pancreas that reduces glucose levels in our blood, is released into the blood as soon as the body detects that blood sugar levels have risen above their optimal level.

Insulin is a very efficient hormone that runs the body's fuel storage systems. If there is excess sugar or fat in the insulin in the blood, it will tell the body to store it in the body's fat cells. Insulin also tells these cells not to release their stored fat, making that fat unavailable for the body to use for energy.

Because this stored fat cannot be released for use as energy, insulin effectively prevents weight loss. The higher the body's insulin levels, the more effectively it will prevent fat cells from releasing their stores, and the harder it will be to lose weight. According to many authorities, in the long term, high levels of insulin can lead to insulin resistance and cause serious health problems such as those listed below:

1. Increased insulin levels and insulin resistance
2. Decreased metabolism leading to weight gain
3. Increase in fat tissue and reduction in muscle tissue
4. Accelerated aging
5. Increased food allergies and intolerances
6. Overburdened immune system
7. Increased risk of heart disease, obesity, diabetes, and cancer

Carbohydrates, especially simple carbohydrates such as sugar and starch, quickly become sucrose through the body and enter the bloodstream faster, causing the release of large amounts of insulin. The fewer carbohydrates you eat, the less insulin your body produces, and the fewer calories you store as fat. Less fat storage means less weight gain and fewer carbohydrates consumed means less insulin in the blood and in the body that uses its fat reserves as fuel.

The premise behind every low-carb diet plan is that a body that produces less insulin burns more fat than a body that produces a lot of insulin. Some plans encourage an extremely low carbohydrate intake period so that the body enters a state of ketosis and burns fat deposits more quickly.

These are usually called induction periods. The duration of extreme carbohydrate control ranges from seven days to the time it takes you to reach your ideal weight. After this period of extremely low-carbohydrate diet, maintenance levels of carbohydrate intake are followed to prevent weight gain. The amount of carbohydrates you can safely eat will depend on your unique body system. And you'll probably have to experiment to figure out what level of carbohydrate intake is best for you.

No matter what your carbohydrate intake, it will be lower than normal and still eliminate white flour and white flower products and certain other sugary and starchy foods. This is why these diet plans are known as low-carbohydrate lifestyles.

Low-carbohydrate success requires that you be willing to stop consuming simple carbohydrates in the long run.

Now, here's a list of the most popular low-carb diet plans and books and a summary of their requirements.

14 Most Popular and Effective Diets: Atkins Diet

Perhaps the most widely known of all low-carbohydrate diets is the Atkins diet. Created by Dr. Robert Atkins in the 1970s, the Atkins diet is considered by some to be the most extreme low-carbohydrate diet plan.

Dr. Atkins believed that almost all obesity is caused by the production of overactive insulin and not by overeating. He believed that excess food could be caused by carbohydrate addiction and that most overweight people actually ate less than their thin counterparts. However, they crave and eat carbohydrates, which increases their insulin levels and suppresses fat burning.

Dr. Atkins is an advocate of ketogenic fat burning, which is achieved by eating less than 40 grams of carbohydrates each day. He advises his followers to buy test strips so that they can measure the amount of ketones in their urine daily and confirm that they are in a constant state of ketosis. It also recommends the use of dietary supplements to help balance nutrition and the body's systems.

The Atkins diet is divided into four stages: the induction diet, the continuous weight loss diet, the pre-maintenance diet, and finally the lifelong maintenance diet.

The induction diet is very strict in terms of elimination of carbohydrates (20 grams or less per day), but generous in terms of the amount of fat and protein. It should be noted that low starch vegetables are the recommended source of carbohydrates. This phase of the diet lasts 14 days and is followed by the Continuous Weight Loss (OWL) diet.

The OWL phase allows for the reintroduction of certain good carbohydrates, but levels remain below 40 grams per day. Dieters stay on OWL until they reach their ideal weight. Once the ideal weight is reached, dieters move on to the Pre-Maintenance diet, where they experiment with reintroducing certain good carbohydrates until they discover their level of carbohydrate tolerance (the total number of grams of carbohydrates they can consume in a day and not gain weight).

When dieters understand the amount of carbohydrates they can consume and maintain their ideal weight, they enter the lifetime maintenance program. Here they will continue to avoid sugar, processed foods, white flour, and hydrogenated oils and fats.

The Atkins diet offers a number of approved foods and there are Atkins stores in many areas that sell diet-compatible products.

> ### *The Diet of Carbohydrate Addicts*

Rachael and Richard Heller introduced the term "carbohydrate addict" in their 1993 book The Carbohydrates Addict's Diet.

The idea is that some people are addicted to carbohydrates just as alcoholics are addicted to alcohol and drug addicts are addicted to drugs. This addiction causes strong cravings, insulin resistance, and weight gain.

Dr. Rachael Heller developed the diet to eliminate her own obesity and had maintained her dramatic weight loss for over twenty years when the first book was written. Heller's believes that the insulin imbalance caused by carbohydrates causes the body to crave more food and interferes with the release of serotonin, which would indicate that the body is full. This leads to overeating and weight gain.

Heller's recommends that the carbohydrate addict limit his carbohydrate intake to a "reward meal," eat three times a day and avoid snacks until the person is out of the weight-loss phase of the diet.

In addition to the diet plan, Heller's also

cover psychological triggers that can cause carbohydrate addicts to binge on carbohydrates and gain weight. Dieters are encouraged to identify personal emotional triggers and how to avoid these triggers to help lose weight.

One of the most important theories of this diet is that overweight is not the fault of the obese person. Why is that? Because the biology of the person and the addictive power of carbohydrates is working against them.

Like all other low-carbohydrate plans, Heller recommends avoiding processed foods and many types of sugar. However, they also state that some starchy carbohydrates should be consumed with reward meals if desired, so that the dieter is more likely to follow the long-term diet.

Heller's believe that carbohydrate addiction is treated long term with good nutrition and a proper diet, but it is never cured and carbohydrate addicts should be vigilant to prevent future weight gain and carbohydrate binge eating.

> ### ➢ *The Hampton Diet*

Dr. Fred Pescatore, former Associate Medical Director of the Atkins Institute, developed the Hampton Diet. This diet is a mixture of low-carbohydrate diet concepts and the healthiest concepts of the Mediterranean diet. Encourages liberal consumption of monounsaturated fats to help lose weight and prevent diseases such as cancer, heart disease and diabetes. All of this is set out in The Hampton's Diet, published in May 2004.

His book includes a thirty-day meal

plan, gourmet recipes and information on Australian macadamia nut oil, which he encourages dieters to use abundantly. He suggests the use of special cold pressed virgin olive oil if you can't afford the macadamia nut oil he considers the best for your health.

There are a large number of recipes, but most of them use expensive ingredients and are quite gourmet. World-class chefs and restaurant owners contributed many of the book's recipes to their own successful low-carb creations enjoyed by customers around the world.

Due to Dr. Pescatore's affiliation with Dr. Atkins, his diet is strongly influenced by the Atkins diet. The main points of difference seem to be a greater emphasis on fruits and vegetables, the use of healthier fats such as macadamia nut oil, and the suggestion that all skin and fat be removed from meat before cooking.

This plan has many of the same features as Atkins, but with tasty recipes and 30-day meal plans and more than 100 recipes.

➢ *The Glycemic Index Diet*

Written by Rick Gallop, former president of The Heart and Stroke Foundation of Ontario, The Glycemic Index (GI) Diet states, "If you can understand a traffic light, you will understand this diet.

Galloping divides foods into three groups based on their glycemic index, that is, how quickly they cause increases in blood sugar levels. Separate foods into light green, light yellow and light red. Glucose is set at a GI level of 100 and all other foods are compared to it. Red light foods should be avoided, yellow light foods are avoided during the initial weight loss phase and eaten occasionally during the ongoing maintenance phase and green light foods should form the basis of your diet at all times.

There is no need to buy special foods. Just find out where your favorite foods fit into the plan, eat green, try a little yellow, and avoid red. That's it. Galopar says that dieters should expect to lose one to two pounds per week and don't need to start on a shock diet. While this is a low-carbohydrate diet, it is not as high in protein as most other diets and encourages dieters to reduce fats as well as carbohydrates. It also encourages exercising for 30 minutes each day and eating three balanced meals that include carbohydrates, proteins, and fats.

According to Gallop, followers of the GI diet should consider it a lifestyle change to which they will adhere for the rest of their lives, not a diet. But it's not easy. For example, consider this list of "red light foods" and write down all "good foods:

- Beans cooked with pork Refried beans Alcoholic beverages Regular soft drinks Bagels
- Croissants Baguettes Cake Cookies Cornbread
- English buns Hamburger buns Hot dog buns Kaiser rolls Pancakes Pancakes Waffles
- Pizza
- Regular Granola Bar Filling
- Tortillas White bread Millet
- White rice Instant rice Rice cakes Cold cereals
- Wheat Granola Cream
- Maize semolina Muesli
- Instant Avena Croutons Ketchup Mayonnaise Tartar sauce

Cheese Milk Chocolate Cheese Cottage Cream

-   Cream cheese Ice cream Whole milk/2% Sour cream Yogurt

-   Butter Coconut oil

-   Hard Margarine Butter

-   Palm oil Peanut butter

-   Regular salad dressing Tropical oils

-   Vegetable butter Cantaloupe

-   Dates

-   Melon melon honey Prunes

-   Watermelon with raisins

-   Canned fruit in syrup All dried fruits Sugar apple compote All fruit drinks

-   Prune juice Sorbet Bologna Bratwurst Regular eggs

-   Ground beef burgers with 20% fat

-   Hotdogs Pastrami Processed meat Regular bacon

-   Sausage sausages Sushi rolls

-   All canned pasta Couscous Gnocchi

-   Macaroni with cheese and noodles
-   Pasta stuffed with meat or cheese Alfredo sauces
-   Sauces with Jell-O sugar
-   French fries Candy French fries

➢ *NeanderThin*

Ray Audette, the author of NeanderThin promotes his diet as a way to "eat like a caveman for a slim, strong, healthy body. At the tender age of 33, Audette suffered from rheumatoid arthritis and diabetes. After hearing from doctors that her condition was treatable but not curable, Audette decided to undertake nutritional research to find a better cure.

His research led him to adopt a "paleolithic" hunter-gatherer diet, like the one our human ancestors ate before settling into agrarian societies. Within a week, her blood sugar levels were normal and after a month she had lost 25 pounds, her arthritic pain was relieved and she noticed an improvement in muscle tone.

According to Audette, our Palaeolithic ancestors were much healthier and lived longer than our Neolithic agrarian ancestors. He claims that the Neolithic man was shorter, had poorer dental health, and was more prone to obesity than the Paleolithic man. Women also began menstruating earlier and having more children together, leading to an increase in the population that further encouraged agrarian lifestyles.

It suggests that modern man should become a modern hunter-gatherer by eliminating foods that need human intervention to be edible. These foods include milk, grains, beans, potatoes, alcohol, and sugar. Grains include all wheat, corn, rice, oats, barley, and rye. He also subscribes to the theory that these carbohydrates produce cravings and warns that if consumed they will cause possible binge eating.

The general rule of Audette is that if a fruit or vegetable is unprocessed raw edible, then it is safe on the NeanderThin diet. Explain that many vegetables, such as potatoes, are actually poisonous if not properly stored and treated with fungicides. In addition, it encourages eating fruits when they are in season and limiting winter fruit intake to help the body burn stored fat.

He gives the Ten Commandments. They're condensed:

Eat: meats and fish, fruits, vegetables, nuts and seeds, berries Don't eat: grains, beans, potatoes, dairy, and sugar.

> ## *The Power of Protein*

Drs. Michael and Mary Eades, co-authors of The Protein Power LifePlan, have similar views to Audette and also believe that modern health problems are caused by our modern diet that is heavy on grains and processed foods (Note that Dr. Michael Eades even wrote the introduction to Audette's NeanderThin).

The Eades offer a food pyramid that is the USDA pyramid upside down, so protein forms the base, vegetables and fruits form the center, and whole grains form the tip of the pyramid.

In addition to basing their diet on high protein and low grain intake, Eades also encourage regular exercise and modify regular tanning without sunscreen to help the body produce the necessary vitamins and regulate body systems. They also recommend taking a complete multivitamin and mineral supplement daily.

Dieters should identify their minimum protein requirements per meal by height, weight, and sex. Each meal should include at least the amount of protein and protein that should be consumed at each meal. Dieters should eliminate bad fats, which include corn oil, vegetable cooking oils, margarine, vegetable shortening, and all partially hydrogenated oils.

The diet can be followed in phases that allow for a rapid transition to low-carbohydrate and accelerated weight loss. The first phase is called Intervention and carbohydrate intake is limited to 7 to 10 grams per meal. The second phase is called the transition level and must be completed over several months. At this level up to 15 net grams of carbohydrates per meal are allowed. In the final maintenance phase, up to 30 grams of carbohydrates can be consumed with each meal. In addition, they offer food choices and plans for 3 types of low-carbohydrate diets: Purists, Hedonists and Dilettantes.

Purists seek to replicate a Palaeolithic style of eating in the modern world and will rely heavily on animal proteins and will avoid all dairy products, alcohol, caffeine, legumes, sugars (except honey), processed foods, grain cereals and products containing them. In addition, they will eat fresh and organic fruits and vegetables and natural or game meat products.

Hedonists are allowed the greatest

freedom of action in the diet. They simply need to consume enough protein, keep carbohydrates within the limits set for each meal, consume plenty of water and good fats, and take potassium and magnesium supplements.

The Dilettantes walk the middle way between these two extremes. They continue to avoid wheat, maize, millet, rye and products produced from their flours. However, they are allowed carbohydrates within daily guidelines, some natural sugars and organic dairy products.

> ***Principle of Schwarzbein***
-

Dr. Diana Schwarzbein is the endocrinologist of the stars. The physician chosen by Suzanne Somers, Larry Hagman and many others, Schwarzbein encourages extensive testing for hormonal imbalances and then suggests several diet and exercise programs and selective hormone replacement to treat any deficiency.

The principles of Dr. Schwarzbein's diet are set out in the Schwarzbein Principle, her 5-step plan for optimal health.

The first step in the program is Healthy Nutrition and there are ten basic rules:

1. Never skip a meal again

2. Eat real, unprocessed food

3. Eat balanced meals

4. Choose a protein as the main nutrient in your meal

5. Add some healthy fats

6. Add real carbohydrates

7. Add starch-free vegetables

8. Eating snacks

9. Eat solid foods

10. Drink enough water

The second step in the program is stress management:

1. Make downtime a daily practice

2. Put Your Life in Perspective

3. Stay on top of signs of stress

4. Getting enough sleep

Third, avoid all toxic chemicals, including:

1. Nicotine

2. Alcohol

3. Refined sugar

4. Artificial sweeteners

5. Illegal drugs

6. Monosodium glutamate, additives and preservatives

7. False greases and grease blockers

8. Caffeine

9. Certain prescription drugs

Fourth, practice cardiovascular, endurance, and flexibility/relaxation exercises.

And finally, the fifth step toward optimal health is to take hormone replacement therapy as needed.

Suzanne Somers first introduced "Somersizing" in Suzanne Somers Eat Great, Lose Weight in 1992. Somersizing is a way of eating in which you cut sugar and "funky foods" and eat lots of fats, proteins and good carbohydrates such as vegetables and fruits. Foods must be combined in certain ways for the body to digest them easily. People who do Somersize diet in two steps, the first (Level One) to lose weight and induce "melting" of fat and the second (Level Two) for the ongoing maintenance of their ideal weight.

Somers separates foods into four food groups of Somersizing size: Proteins/Fats, Vegetables, Carbohydrates and Fruits. She suggests the fruit be eaten on an empty stomach. Proteins/fats include meat, plate, eggs, natural oils, butter, cream and cheese. Vegetables include low starch fresh vegetables. Carbos covers whole-grain breads, pastas and cereals, and fat-free dairy products.

List "Seven Easy Steps to Somersizing:

1. Eliminate all funky food.

2. East fruit alone, on an empty stomach: 20 minutes before a Carbos meal, 1 hour before a Pro/Fats meal and at least 2 hours before the last meal of the day.

3. Eat Pro/Fat with Vegetables.

4. Eat carbohydrates with vegetables.

5. Keep Pro/Fats and Carbos separate.

6. Wait 3 hours between meals if you switch from Pro/Fats to Carbos or vice versa.

7. Eat at least 3 meals a day and don't

skip any. Funky Foods include:

White sugar Brown sugar Raw sugar Corn syrup Sucrose Molasses Honey Maple syrup Beetroot Carrots

- Acorn-fed squash Bananas Pumpkin Pumpkin Corn
- Potatoes Parsnips Squashes
- Sweet Potatoes White Flour White Rice
- Yams
- Pumpkin Hubbard Avocados Coconut
- Liver
- Low-fat milk Whole milk nuts
- Olives Soy Beer
- Caffeine Tea Caffeine Cocoa Soda
- Coffee
- Hard Alcohol Wine

All foods on the Funky Foods list should be avoided during the first phase of the diet (Level One), but some may be reintroduced in moderation during the maintenance phase (Level Two). Somers sells its own brand of artificial sweetener called "SomerSweet". All his books include recipes for meals, snacks and desserts.

> ***South Beach Diet***
-

Developed by Dr. Arthur Agatston, the South Beach Diet promotes itself as a way to teach dieters to eat the right carbohydrates and fats. The diet has three phases. In the first diet banish bad carbohydrate cravings and induce rapid weight loss. In the second phase, some types of carbohydrates are reintroduced and weight loss is slower. The final phase is the "Diet for Life" phase. This is the maintenance diet and will be followed for the rest of the life of the person doing the diet. If at any time the dieter begins to gain unwanted weight, then he simply goes through the induction and pre-maintenance phases again.

The first phase emphasizes protein from high-quality meat sources with lots of fresh vegetables and salads with real olive oil dressing. Bread, rice, pasta, potatoes, baked goods, soy milk and cheese, yogurt, beets, carrots, corn and all fruit are prohibited in the 14-day induction phase. This includes all sweets, cakes, ice cream, and sugar, plus meats that are cured with sugar or molasses.

The diet encourages three meals a day with a mid-morning snack and a mid-afternoon snack.

There is also a daily meal plan. This plan includes a strict control of the portions in the induction phase. An example of a daily snack is 20 peanuts. And 30 pistachios is another sandwich option.

Unlike Atkins, unlimited protein intake is not recommended or allowed in this diet. However, during the later stages of the diet, some of the strict portion controls end and dieters can eat until they are satiated.

Some of the banned foods can be reintroduced slowly, sometimes in modified form in the second phase of the diet. The second phase lasts until the target weight of the dieter is reached. However, white flour products, potatoes, maize, carrots, beet and sweet fruits such as bananas and pineapples are still banned.

After dieters reach their ideal weight,

they move on to their lifetime diet or maintenance diet.

In this phase the prohibited foods are processed foods, white flour products, sweet fruits and foods with a high glycemic index in general.

During the 14-day induction period, Dr. Agatston predicts a weight loss of between 8 and 13 pounds, with abdominal fat being the first to disappear. In the second phase the dieter should continue to lose 1 to 2 pounds each week as long as it is not exceeded with the reintroduction of carbohydrates.

> ***Lucky hunter!***

At Sugar Busters! dieters cut sugar to reduce fat. This diet was created by a group of doctors and the CEO of a New Orleans Fortune 500 business who realized that low-fat foods are full of sugar and that it is the sugar in foods that produces a negative insulin response and leads to weight gain.

They emphasize the enjoyment of good food and avoid certain banned foods such as processed sugar and refined grain products. Sugar is not prohibited, but overtime consumption of sugar should be significantly reduced, and dieters should begin to recognize products with hidden sugars. The right combination of foods to help prevent weight gain is also emphasized.

This plan eliminates potatoes, corn, white flour, white rice, refined flour bread, most cold cereals, beets, carrots, refined sugar, corn syrup, molasses, honey, sugared colas and beer.

The authors also recommend eating fruits alone and eating whole fruits as much as possible. They allow for three meals, two snacks, and one sugar-free dessert, but the emphasis is on being able to control food portions, similar to what fits comfortably on a normal-sized plate.

The diet begins with a 14-day diet plan and includes a meal planner. Dieters are advised to eat carbohydrates high in fiber and low in starch that have a lower glycemic index. The authors also encourage the consumption of lean, well-cut meats for protein. They estimate that you will consume about 30 percent protein, 40 percent carbohydrates, and 30 percent monounsaturated oils and other fats.

> ***The Zone***

Created by Dr. Barry Sears, The Zone encourages balanced consumption of carbohydrates and proteins. Dr. Sears suggests that you divide your plate into three sections, one for protein and two for fruits and vegetables per meal. This results in 30 percent protein, 40 percent carbohydrates and 30 percent fat. For each meal, the protein portion should be about the size of your tightly clenched fist. The carbohydrate portion should be the size of two clenched fists and the added fat portion should be about the volume of your thumb.

The Zone is all about measuring and controlling food portions. Another tool that dieters in the Zone can use to measure food is the "block. Each adult is allowed at least 11 blocks per day and the proper size of the food portion will affect the amount of food per volume that a dieter actually consumes each day.

This plan does not allow unlimited servings of protein or eating until you are satiated. Once the food portions in your Zone are gone, your food will be ready.

The basic rules of the Zone are:

1. Eat a Zone meal within an hour after waking up each day.
2. Eat a balanced meal from the Zone each time you eat (protein, carbohydrates, fat).
3. Eat five times a day; three meals, two snacks.
4. Never go more than five hours without eating a local meal.
5. Eat more fruits and vegetables and bread, pasta, grains, and starches.

6. Drink 64 ounces of water a day.

7. If you make a mistake at one meal, make your next meal friendly to the area.

Although foods are not prohibited in the Zone diet, certain unfavorable carbohydrates should be avoided or, if eaten, do not constitute more than 25 percent of any food or snack. Unfavourable carbohydrates are the usual suspects: white flour, potatoes, sugar, white rice, juices, soft drinks, alcohol, bananas, grapes, carrots, corn and caffeinated beverages. Dr. Sears believes that these foods not only increase insulin production, but can also cause hormonal imbalances and inflammation of body tissues, leading to illness and overall poor health.

The Zone's diet also includes packaged

foods such as nutritional bars, beverages, bakery products and nutritional supplements. But be careful, the Zone nutrition bar contains high fructose corn syrup, but according to the website, it's a very "high quality" type that has a slower glycemic index than the common type, and the protein in the bar helps further delay insulin response. Use with extreme caution.

> ## *Slim forever*

Before he began extolling the virtues of Australian macadamia nut oil, Dr. Fred Pescatore wrote the book Thin For Good: The Only Low-Carbohydrate Diet That Will Finally Work for You. This plan explores the mind-body connection in lasting weight loss and includes plans for men and women, as well as a low-carbohydrate diet plan for vegetarians.

In Thin For Good, Dr. Pescatore presents "The Eleven Emotional Levels of Food" that they are:

1 Anger: often feels at the beginning of a new diet, or ourselves for gaining weight; but this is good because it is motivating.

2 Frustration: may be the result of looking at the success of others and comparing it to our apparent lack of success; but be careful - this is a negative emotion and often the one that makes people give up.

3 Sadness: closely linked to self-pity or mourning for old ways of life and food.

4 Fear: this emotion is often very difficult to let go and usually appears at the same time as the first successes in weight loss (Can I keep this diet for the rest of my life?)

5 Understanding: you must work through the first 4 emotions to get to this more positive point when you begin to understand what your bad eating habits are and accept them.

6 Trepidation: described as nervousness, nervousness and suspicion; the doubt that can arise as you begin to see the results of your diet.

7 Envy: a harmful emotion that arises when compared to others

8 Boredom: this emotion can kill a diet;

add some variety to your meals according to your diet plan.

9 Relief: the beginning of positive emotions to be enjoyed 10 Joy: comes after you have achieved real results; try not to sabotage it with negative thoughts

11 Content: the final emotion experienced once people realize their weight loss goals.

Along with various exercises to help you work through your emotions, Dr. Pescatore suggests low-carbohydrate comfort food recipes that, he says, can help you feel better about dealing with these emotions.

He suggests "Mind Over Calories" as a concept to embrace because it will help you maintain weight forever. He reveals that this concept helped him once he lost weight and has helped him maintain it. The mind about calories is about training yourself not to crave sugary, bad tasting carbohydrate foods that will ruin your life.

It also includes suggestions for dietary supplements for men and women, foods to avoid if you are on a diet restricted by yeasts, have hormonal or thyroid problems, and more than 40 pages of recipes.

An additional advantage is the Thin For Good Food pyramid which has proteins and fats in the body.

> ***The 7-day low-carbohydrate rescue and recovery plan***

This book was written by Drs. Rachel and Richard Heller and is promoted as the book for anyone with a low-carbohydrate diet on any plan that needs help getting back on track - right now.

This is the book for the person who has let a vacation, a vacation or a bad choice of spiral food into a crisis or who are discouraged because they have reached a plateau of unwanted weight loss.

Doctors offer a 7-day meal plan to help you get back to normal, as well as tips for curbing your carbohydrate cravings, dealing with saboteurs, and identifying hidden carbohydrates and sugars.

First, the Hellers explain that overweight people and those with sweet teeth are physiologically different from naturally thin people and need to stop blaming themselves for their weight problems. Understanding what your body needs - and what you need to avoid - to lose weight will only help you reach your goals sooner.

The 7-day diet plan they propose helps rebalance insulin levels, curb cravings and put the body back into fat-burning mode. Once this is done, you can return to your low-carbohydrate plan with new insights on how to avoid the most common dangers. There are 7 steps, which are added one each day. They are:

1. Add a low-carb protein to every meal and snack
2. Add low-carb vegetables and/or salads to lunch, dinner, and snacks.

3. Include a good portion of low-carbohydrate protein, vegetables and/or salads in relation to the high-carbohydrate foods you may be eating.

4. Eat all of your low-carbohydrate protein, vegetables, and salads before eating your high-carbohydrate meal.

5. Eat only low-carb snacks. Save carbohydrate-rich foods for meals.

6. Eat only low-carbohydrate foods at all snacks and at one meal.

7. Eat only low-carbohydrate foods at all snacks and at two meals.

After successfully completing these steps for 7 days, you may return to the low-carbohydrate plan of your choice. They also suggest that you avoid sugar substitutes such as those found in the diet: tails to help you stay on your diet plan.

In addition, everyone with low-carbohydrate content is encouraged to eat towards carbohydrates in their meals. In this way they are first filled with proteins and the lowest starch carbohydrates. Finally, you can eat the highest starch and carbohydrate meal on your plate. This will help you fill up and eat less of the foods that may be causing you problems. In addition, once carbohydrate-rich foods reach your body, they will be so busy breaking down the protein and fiber you ate that you will more slowly digest the bad carbohydrates you consumed.

➢ *Living with low carbohydrate intake*

Written by Fran McCullough, author of The Low-Carb Cookbook, the long subtitle of this book promises to teach "everything dieters need to know to achieve lasting success, including: strategies to control binge drinking and cravings, deal with sudden weight gain, and secret metabolic weapons.

This book is a supplement to the low-carbohydrate diet of your choice and is intended to give you tips and tricks to make the road to low-carbohydrate success smoother and much less hilly.

This volume contains sources of low-carb bread and other products and how to make vegetables taste the same as pasta. There are also tips for various kitchen utensils that can make your life easier and suggestions for storing a low-carbohydrate pantry.

McCullough also offers suggestions for low-carbohydrate eating in a very active lifestyle. For example, there are tips for camping or backpacking in Europe. There are also suggestions for managing your carbohydrate cravings with low-carbohydrate substitutes.

For example, give a simple recipe for a pizza without crust and potato skins. There is even a suggestion of an ice cream substitute that incorporates dairy and fruit.

Although McCullough reviews many of the basic concepts of the low-carbohydrate diet at the beginning of this book, he mainly gives tips, tricks, and recipes. Don't look here for the basics of diet.

Practical tips for success

Dieting is not easy. If it was, we'd probably all be thin. Since we're not, here are some tips that successful people use to lose weight so others can benefit as well.

- **Practical advice: DRINK 8 TO 10 VASES OF WATER PER DAY**

Okay, for a lot of people this is a big problem. Water doesn't taste so good in general because water doesn't really "taste" like anything. Drinking water 8 to 10 times a day is easier the more you do it. It's simply a matter of conditioning your taste buds, and yourself, to make it easier to do.

Once you start, you'll start to crave water.

To start, you should drink a glass of water in the morning first thing in the morning, before you eat. This is probably the easiest glass you will drink all day and will help you remember to drink water all day. Better yet, why not drink two glasses?

If you really can't stand the taste of water, try using a water purifier pitcher or filter. You can also add a few drops of lemon or lime to your water, but without sugar or sweetener. Ice helps, too.

Check out the flavored waters on the market, too. Just be on the lookout for additives.

- ***Practical advice:***
DESAYUNAR

Don't skip breakfast. If you need to go to bed a little earlier so you can get up 20 minutes earlier each morning, do it! Breakfast is very important for your good health and weight control. According to Dr. Barbara Rolls, professor of nutrition at Penn State University, "Your metabolism slows down while you sleep, and it doesn't accelerate until you eat again.

Eating breakfast is not only good for overall weight loss, but it will help you stay on the right track with your diet the rest of the day. You're more likely to be attracted to something sweet and the "bread" group if you skip breakfast.

You can always keep a couple of hard-boiled eggs in the refrigerator or a little fruit with high fiber and low starch content. If you plan to eat fruit throughout the day, breakfast is the perfect time to do so.

- ***Practical advice: EAT AT LEAST 3 MEALS AND 2 REFRIGERATIONS EVERY DAY***

This can be one of the most difficult adjustments to make. After all, you're busy! You already have a full plate. When do you have time to worry about filling your plate with more frequent meals?

Just as breakfast will increase your metabolism, it will also make you eat more often. This will also help you reduce your intake of bad carbohydrates by making sure your snacks are planned and occur regularly throughout the day.

In reality, it only takes a minimal investment of planning time at the grocery store and at home each morning before you leave each day to make some healthy food choices and prepare some healthy snacks and meals. For suggestions, just see the list of snacks and appetizers below.

- ***Practical advice: AVOID WHITE FOODS***

This is an easy way to remember what not to eat. If it's made of sugar, flour, potatoes, rice or corn, just say no. Remembering this rule of thumb will make it easier to recognize these rice cakes as an unhealthy, high-carbohydrate snack.

Always look for colorful fruits and

vegetables to replace white ones. Buy broccoli, lettuce, peppers, green beans and peas, brown rice in moderation, green leafy vegetables such as kale and spinach, apples, melons, oranges and grapes.

These foods are not only colorful, but also high in fiber, nutrients, and important antioxidants. Eating colorful fruits and vegetables will add variety to your diet, as well as additional health benefits.

- ***Practical advice: EAT YOUR VEGETABLES***

It is so easy to use a low-carbohydrate diet as an excuse for poor nutrition. Resist this temptation. If the only vegetable you've eaten in the last 5 years has been the potato, now is a good time to start experimenting with other vegetables. This is important for your overall health and to avoid some unpleasant side effects of not getting enough fiber in your diet.

   If you try hard enough, you'll find vegetables you'll like to eat. Experiment with grilled vegetables and cook with real butter for flavor. You can also search for new recipes on the Internet or in cookbooks.

   Remember, if you're only eating 40 grams of carbohydrates a day or less, two cups of green salads contain only about 5 grams of carbohydrates. You have no excuse not to eat your vegetables.

- ***Practical advice: PREPARE YOUR OWN FOOD AS MUCH AS POSSIBLE***

While more and more restaurants offer

low-carbohydrate dishes, many of them are still not the best choice. There are many recipes for a quick

and easy meals that you can prepare yourself at home. Try to do this as often as possible.

If you cook your own foods, you know exactly what the content is and can better control hidden sugar and processed foods in another way.

Another advantage is long-term cost savings. Even if you have to go to the grocery store more often, you will save a significant amount per meal instead of eating in restaurants and fast food establishments.

It will also be easier to keep your diet

with your own favorite fresh food
selections on hand.

> ● ***Practical advice: INVEST IN
> A GOOD SET OF FOOD STORAGE
> CELLS***

Having food storage containers of
various sizes on hand will make planning
your meals and snacks much easier. When
you buy nuts, fruits and vegetables in
bulk, you can simply prepare them,
separate them and store them for easy
use later.

For example, you can pre-cut apples
and snacks for several days. Simply cut
them, rinse them with pineapple or lemon
juice and put them away. This will be a
quick and easy snack for later.

Prepare your lunch and take it with you to work. Better yet, prepare your lunch and two sandwiches for work.

- ***Practical advice: EAT SOMETHING PROTECTED IN EVERY FOOD AND AS TENTEMPIE***

In addition to everything discussed above, eating protein helps you burn more calories. Jeff Hample, Ph.D., R.D., a spokesman for the American Dietetic Association says, "Protein is composed primarily of amino acids, which are harder for your body to break down, so you burn more calories to get rid of them.

Just think - eating a protein-rich snack can help you lose weight. How about a few slices of turkey or ham or a little shredded cheese?

Eating protein will also help you feel full, so you're less likely to crave an unhealthy snack.

- ***Practical advice: DRINK ONE GLASS OF WATER AFTER EACH BOCADILLO***

This will help you drink 8 to 10 glasses of water a day, but may also have other benefits. Have you ever felt hungry after eating a handful or standard portion of nuts? Try drinking water later. Water will help you feel full and prevent overcomplacency.

Drinking water after a snack will also help take the taste out of your mouth.and can help curb your desire for more.

- ***Practical advice: EAT SLOWLY AND ENJOY FOOD***

You will feel fuller and more satisfied if you take the time to savor your food and chew it more slowly. Don't get used to eating while standing or eating fast. Sit down and chew.

Eating slower will help you enjoy your food more, pay attention to what you're really eating, and get a better idea of when it's full.

- ***Practical advice: EAT THE LARGEST MEALS EARLY AND THE SMALLEST AT THE LATEST.***

You'll feel better and lose weight faster if you have a big breakfast and a smaller dinner. You may also want to eat most of your carbohydrates earlier in the day, saving a salad and lean meat protein for dinner.

Eating larger meals during the part of the day when you're most active will help you feel full throughout the day and curb unhealthy snack cravings.

- ***Practical advice: CONSIDER SALMON OR HORSE MEAL FOR BREAKFAST***

Yes, this may seem strange, but it is a way to work with Omega-3 fatty acids that are good for you and add some variety to your daily diet. After a few months you may get tired of eating eggs and bacon for breakfast. Substituting fish will give you the healthy fish proteins and fish oils you need.

You can try salmon or mackerel on croquettes for a healthier sausage substitute. Or you can just eat the cold salmon left over the next morning with dill sauce.

- ***Practical advice: USE LECHUGA SHEETS IN PLACE OF BREAD***

This advice may seem a little strange at first, but if you try it, you'll probably love it. Instead of eating breads and buns with their sandwiches and hamburgers, why not try lettuce leaves?

You can make a double cheeseburger with onions, pickles and tomatoes wrapped in a whole leaf of lettuce. Or you can make sandwiches with lettuce instead of tortilla and bread.

This will help increase your good carbohydrate and fiber intake while giving you more variety in your diet.

- ***Practical advice: EAT A FRUIT DESSERTRE***

Okay, we all want a little dessert sometime, but how come you have your dessert and your low-carb diet too? Why not try cheese with fruit slices or berries?

Better yet, why not try the berry cream? Can you even try sweet pineapples or strawberries with cottage cheese?

Berries are sweet and rich in fiber and nutrients and dairy products are rich in protein. If your low-carbohydrate plan allows it, this is a sweet and tasty alternative to the more sugary desserts.

An added benefit is that the protein in dairy products and the fiber in fresh fruit will make these desserts fuller.

- ***Practical advice: GET YOUR FRESH FRUIT WITHOUT EXPRESSING IT***

Fruit juice can be very tempting as a substitute for soft drinks, but how healthy is fruit juice? If you read the labels, you will soon realize that in many of the commercial juices available in your local supermarket there is very little fruit juice.

What you'll find is lots of sugar water and other ingredients. Why not skip the juice and eat a piece of fresh fruit? Not only does fresh fruit contain less sugar than juice, fresh fruit has fiber that is good for you and will help you feel fuller for longer.

- ***Practical advice: BE CAREFUL OF FOOD REPLACEMENT***

New shakes and meal replacement bars come on the market almost every day. These smoothies and bars can be said to be healthy, but almost everyone, including Zone Perfect bars, contains hydrogenated oil and sweeteners.

So be careful. Bars especially can only be slightly healthier than a Snickers candy bar. Occasionally, they may not be so bad for you, but as a general rule, you probably don't want to indulge in a milkshake or a meal replacement bar every day.

- ***Practical advice: IF IT SOUNDS TOO GOOD TO BE TRUE, IT WILL PROBABLY NOT BE.***

Low-carb donuts and muffins? You can find these pre-packaged products with low-carbohydrate labels at your neighborhood grocery store and at many low-carbohydrate lifestyle stores. That doesn't mean you should make a habit of eating them.

Although low-carbohydrate cakes can be tempting, remember that they still contain all the usual suspicious carbohydrates: sugar or a sugar and flour substitute.

They may be healthier than typical muffins as an occasional treat, but remember to follow the basic tips for continuing low-carbohydrate success.

• *Practical advice:* *SUPERMARKET*

It's easier to stick to your low-carb lifestyle if you learn the common thread in all grocery store designs: healthy foods are in the perimeter aisles.

Think about it, when you go to the grocery store, all the healthy things, fruits, vegetables, meats and dairy products are arranged around the walls of the stores.

It is rarely necessary to enter the central aisle areas of the few stores that store butter and cheese in the center, near frozen foods. For most of all the foods you need for your low-carbohydrate diet can be found on the perimeter of the grocery store.

Train yourself to start at one end of the outer aisle and work your way. It will be much easier to avoid carbohydrate cravings and fill your basket with healthy items if you do.

- *Practical advice: INVEST IN GOOD KITCHEN BOOKS*

Don't you know what to eat? Does he need variety in his diet? Look for a cookbook. Of course, not every recipe in a cookbook is low-carb, but you'll be amazed at how many low-carb and low-carb recipes you can find in your standard Betty Crocker cookbook.

Cookbooks are excellent reference tools that often contain practical tips for buying meat cuts and preparing meats, fruits and vegetables in new and exciting ways.

In addition, the new low-carb cookbooks are on the market all the time. So be sure to take advantage of these resources to try something new, different and delicious.

- ***Practical advice: TAKE A GOOD MULTIVITAMINIC***

We can't all get it right all the time. Even the most conscientious food blender can lose some healthy vitamins, minerals and trace elements in their diets. To make sure you get everything you need, consider taking a good multivitamin.

Consult your doctor first for recommendations and you should be tested for anemia to see if you need a vitamin with iron. However, the longer you eat low-carbohydrate and the more red meat you eat, the less anemia will be a problem and you will be able to take vitamins with less iron.

Your success is entirely up to you. Assuming you're a healthy individual, your body will do its part. Just remember to stick to the low-carb diet plan that's right for you and add some variety to your meals to help you stay true to your health and weight loss goals.

Recipes and meal ideas

One of the challenges of low-carbohydrate diets is that it's often hard to find appetizing, inexpensive snack options. This is especially true if you have a limited budget and cannot afford to buy special prepackaged foods. Another obstacle to preparing low-carbohydrate snacks and meals is finding ingredients that are appetizing and won't leave you bored after a few days.

Low-carbohydrate dieters need to be creative in their food choices. It's easy to concentrate on foods that aren't allowed. Too often, food that is not allowed seems to be our primary target. However, there are many possibilities for fast food and snacks in front of our eyes if we think of them creatively.

Certain foods are suitable for snacking and also as a basis for a hearty meal. For example, chicken. Chicken breast can be grilled and eaten with several low starch and high fiber vegetables for a nutritious dinner. Cold sliced chicken breasts can also be an appetizing race snack. Here are some ideas for quick meals and take-away snacks.

Make sure your selections are compatible with the low-carbohydrate plan of your choice and are allowed at your plan stage. Enjoy these foods alone as snacks or as part of a main course:

Aperitifs and snacks

- ✓ CHEESE GRAPES IN STRIPS OF APPLES
- ✓ DRIED FRUIT TUNA CANNED CHICKEN CANNED
- ✓ SHRIMP PROSCUITTO WITH COCKTAIL SAUCE
- ✓ ORANGES
- ✓ CELERY STICKS AND EDAMAME PEANUT BUTTER (SOYBEANS)
- ✓ CHICKPEAS HUMMUS
- ✓ HARD-BOILED EGGS LOW-FAT YOGURT
- ✓ SUGAR-FREE APPLE SAUCE LOW-FAT MILK
- ✓ CARROTS SLICED TURKEY CHERRY TOMATOES
- ✓ CUCUMBER WITH SUGAR-FREE DRESSING / SLICED FROZEN BELL PEPPER

✓ ROAST BEEF FRÍO
✓ SARDINES PORK SHELLS
CECINA OYSTERS BACON STRIPS

FRUIT FUN

✓ 1 ½ cups strawberry juice or crushed strawberries
✓ ½ cup orange juice
✓ ¼ cup grapefruit juice
✓ 1 tablespoon lemon juice
✓ 1½ cups of bottled (or tap) water
✓ 1 lb. frozen white grapes (seeded)

Mix all contents in a large pitcher, except grapes. Use frozen grapes as ice cubes; pour and serve.

TASTY TOMATO DELIGHT

✓ 2 cups tomato or vegetable juice 2 tablespoons lemon juice

✓ 1 teaspoon Worcestershire sauce

✓ ½ teaspoon horseradish

✓ A couple of drops of our favorite hot sauce.

Ice cube tray filled with water, sprinkled with drops of lemon juice in each ice cube slot

Place the ice cube tray in the freezer to settle and make lemon-flavored ice cubes. Combine all other ingredients in a pitcher. Stir and serve over lemon ice cubes.

WHIPPED GELATINE TREATMENT

✓ 1 packet sugar-free gelatin, your favorite variety 2/3 cup boiling water

✓ 2 cups of ice cubes

✓ 1 bowl frozen whipped topping, thawed Favourite nuts to taste

Dissolve the gelatine in boiling water. Pour into mixing bowl. Add ice cubes and stir until ingredients thicken. Remove any remaining ice chips.

Mix with whipped cream and stir vigorously until smooth. Serve with a spoon on plates. Decorate with your favorite nuts on top.

- ✓ <font color=#38B0DE>-=½=- Proudly Presents
- ✓ 1 teaspoon cinnamon
- ✓ <font color="#ffff00">-=½=- sync:ßÇÈâÈâ
- ✓ ¼ cup brown sugar
- ✓ TASTY PECANS

Heat oven to 350 degrees. Roasted pecans 10 minutes.

In a mixing bowl, combine: cinnamon, brown sugar, and margarine. Pour over roasted walnuts. Place nuts on a baking sheet and bake for 10 minutes on each side, turning once.

MUSHROOM AND ASPARAGUS OMELETTE

- ✓ 2 eggs
- ✓ 2 tablespoons water
- ✓ 3 stalks of fresh asparagus, stalk removed
- ✓ ¼ cup sliced white mushrooms
- ✓ ¼ cup shredded low-fat mozzarella cheese

Spray small skillet with nonstick oil spray and heat over medium heat. Beat the eggs and water lightly (by hand is good). Pour water-egg mixture into skillet.

When the top is firm, spoon the asparagus, mushrooms and cheese into

half of the tortilla. Double the other half.
Serve.

BROCCOLI WITH CHEESE AND GARLIC

- ✓ 1 pound broccoli flowers 2 cloves garlic, chopped
- ✓ 2 tablespoons extra virgin olive oil
- ✓ ¼ cup shredded fresh cheese (your favorite type)

Steam broccoli in 2 inches of water for 2 minutes. Drain. Heat olive oil in a skillet over medium heat, stirring to cover bottom of skillet. Add garlic and sauté until fragrant (about 1 minute).

Add broccoli and sauté for about 4 minutes, stirring often. Remove skillet from heat. Sprinkle cheese over broccoli. Slight shake.

ALMONDS WITH BUTTER AND GREEN BEANS

- ✓ 1 pound green beans 3 tablespoons butter
- ✓ ½ cup chopped almonds salt and pepper to taste

Cook the green beans in a little salted water for about 5 minutes. Drain. In a skillet, sauté almonds in butter for 2 minutes, stirring frequently. Add green beans and sauté for another 2 minutes, stirring frequently.

CREAMY CAULIFLOWER

- ✓ 1 pound cauliflower bouquets
- ✓ ¼ cup grated cheese (Parmesan or your favorite)
- ✓ ¼ cup whipped cream 1 tablespoon soft butter
- ✓ ¼ teaspoon salt
- ✓ 1/8 teaspoon pepper

Steam cauliflower in 2 inches of water for about 18 minutes or until tender. Add water if necessary during steam cooking). Drain.

In a blender or food processor, puree cauliflower. Add other ingredients. Mix lightly. Place on a covered plate and refrigerate. Can be reheated over low heat.

MEAT BALLS

- ✓ ½ pound ground pork 1 pound ground chicken
- ✓ 1 small onion, finely chopped 1 egg
- ✓ 2 cloves garlic, minced 2 tablespoons minced dill
- ✓ 2 tablespoons canola oil
- ✓ salt and pepper to taste

✓ Preheat oven to 375 degrees.
In a bowl, mix all ingredients
EXCEPT oil.

✓ Good together. Make about 12
meatballs with the mixture.

Heat oil in a skillet over medium heat
and brown meatballs. Transfer skillet (or
place meatballs on cookie sheet or baking
sheet) and bake for 15 minutes or until
fully cooked.

LIST OF JOES

✓ 1 pound ground beef
✓ 2 tablespoons chopped onion
salt and pepper to taste
✓ ½ teaspoon garlic
✓ 1 cup crushed tomatoes
✓ 3 tablespoons brown sugar
✓ 1 teaspoon Worcestershire
sauce
✓ low-carbohydrate (or at least
anything but white!) buns or lettuce
leaves

Brown the meat and drain it. Reduce fire to low. Add the rest of the ingredients. Cook slowly for about 10 minutes and serve on whole wheat or multigrain rolls or lettuce leaves.

STUFFED CHICKEN

- ✓ 4 boneless, skinless chicken breasts (divided in two) Parmesan cheese (to sprinkle to taste)
- ✓ 1 ½ cups chopped mushrooms 1 cup chicken broth
- ✓ 2 tablespoons roasted red pepper, chopped 1 tablespoon water
- ✓ 1 clove garlic, minced
- ✓ ¼ teaspoon dried marjoram, crushed 1 teaspoon cooking oil

Make the filling by combining mushrooms, garlic, pepper and marjoram in a skillet sprayed with fat-free cooking spray. Finish when the mushrooms are tender.

Make an opening in the chicken pieces to create a pocket. Stuff with the stuffing you just made and sprinkle the inside pocket with cheese. (If desired, close with toothpicks).

Brown chicken on both sides in a skillet, cooking in oil. Add the broth. Cook over medium-low heat until chicken is no longer pink inside. Serve with broth poured over the chicken.

Conclusion

I just want to tell you this:

Just remember that everything will not happen overnight and that it will take time before you see a change in your life for the better.

Now yes, I wish you the best in your results, and remember, everything is practical; theory without action is of no use to you. It brings everything you learn into real life.

A big hug, your friend, Jessy!

By the way, when you achieve your

results little by little, I highly recommend you, if you want to learn much more about methods of losing weight, I highly recommend you, my book, on "HOW TO LOSE 10 BOOKS OF WEIGHT IN 10 DAYS QUICKLY", is a book that I'm sure will help you a lot on your way to "good health". Without further ado, you can find it in the Amazon search engine, like: "How to lose 10 pounds of weight in 10 days quickly" or looking for my name, like: "Jessy M. Brown"... Once again I wish you success in your results!